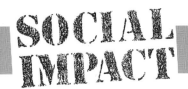
SOCIAL IMPACT

Drugs and Sports

Katherine S. Talmadge
Illustrated by Larry Raymond

TWENTY-FIRST CENTURY BOOKS
FREDERICK, MARYLAND

Published by
Twenty-First Century Books
38 South Market Street
Frederick, Maryland 21701

Printed in the United States of America

10 9 8 7 6 5 4 3 2

Library of Congress Cataloging in Publication Data

Talmadge, Katherine
Drugs and Sports
Illustrated by Larry Raymond

(A Social Impact Book)
Includes glossary and index.
Summary: Discusses the unwise mixing of drugs and sports,
including the stories of several athletes who know the
pain of drug use and addiction.
1. Doping in sports—Juvenile literature.
[1. Drug abuse. 2. Doping in sports.]
I. Raymond, Larry, ill. II. Title.
III. Series: The Social Impact Series.
RC1230.T35 1991
362.29'08'8796—dc20 90-25439 CIP AC
ISBN 0-941477-59-2

Contents

Preface

This book contains the stories of athletes. Some of the athletes mentioned or quoted in this book have used drugs. And they have seen their lives changed because of drugs. Some have even become addicted to drugs. But it should be pointed out that other athletes who are mentioned or quoted have never used drugs. Their comments are included here because they have valuable things to say about the problem of drugs and sports. Just because they appear in this book does not mean that they have been drug users.

Sadly, many athletes—both male and female—have, in fact, turned to drugs. You will notice, as you read, that I use the word "he" many times to refer to an athlete. By doing this, I don't mean to say that all important athletes are men. Certainly, this is not true. But, of course, most of the athletes in the major professional sports are men, and that is why I have so often used the word "he."

I am very grateful for the help that I received as I wrote this book. First, I would like to thank Jeffrey Shulman, at Twenty-First Century Books, for his guidance. My friends and colleagues Susan DeStefano and Pierre Sallé helped with suggestions, corrections, and encouragement. And, finally, I want to thank the athletes themselves, particularly John Lucas and Derek Sanderson. These men generously gave me hours of their time and shared often painful details of their lives. They know firsthand the pain of drug use and addiction, and they paid heavily for choosing to use drugs as a "solution" to the problems and pressures they faced. They shared their stories with me, and now with you, to help you have stronger, safer, and happier lives.

Please listen to their words carefully.

Say "No" to drugs.

1

Athletes and Drugs

The world of sports is filled with excitement.

It's filled with the excitement of close races, when two people are running neck and neck, straining as hard as they can to get just one step ahead of each other. They are just about to reach the finish line, and in the final second, one of the runners thrusts ahead and wins!

The world of sports is filled with the excitement of close games. It's the bottom of the ninth inning, with the score tied and the league championship on the line. With two strikes against him, your favorite player hits a home run! Your team wins the pennant!

The world of sports is filled with talented people. It's filled with men and women who have worked hard to make their bodies healthy, strong, and fast. It's filled with men and women who have the determination to endure years of training and the courage to face the toughest competition, men and women who have dedicated their lives to being the best athletes they can be.

The world of sports is filled with fun. There's the fun of attending a game, the fun of collecting cards and autographs. There's the fun of pretending to be your favorite sports hero when you play basketball or baseball with your friends.

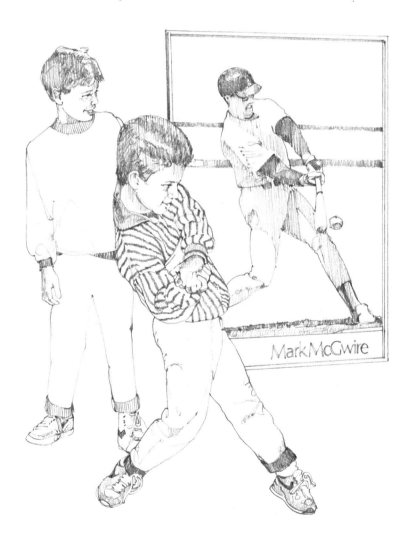

Mark McGwire

But, more and more, the world of sports is filled with something else—something that doesn't belong in sports, something that has hurt the games and the players. It's something that has hurt the fun.

The world of sports is filled with drugs.

- John Lucas was a three-time All-American in basketball at the University of Maryland. In 1976, he was the first draft pick of the National Basketball Association (NBA), and he became one of the best point guards in professional basketball. But he was suspended from three different teams and nearly lost his pro career. Why? Because John Lucas was addicted to cocaine and alcohol.

- At the 1988 Olympic games, sprinter Ben Johnson was forced to return the gold medal he won for his record-breaking time of 9.79 seconds in the 100-meter dash. His time was taken out of the record books, and he was also forbidden from entering any races for a period of two years. Why? Because Ben Johnson had used anabolic steroids.

- Steve Howe, a talented pitcher for the Los Angeles Dodgers and National League Rookie of the Year in 1980, was dropped by the Dodgers in 1985 and then dropped by the minor leagues in 1986. His baseball career was finished. Why? Because Steve Howe was hooked on cocaine.

- Derek Sanderson, who was the National Hockey League (NHL) Rookie of the Year in 1968 and at one time was the highest paid professional athlete in the world, found himself penniless and washed-up as an athlete. Why? Because Derek Sanderson was addicted to alcohol and other drugs.

- Like John Lucas, Len Bias was a basketball star at the University of Maryland. In 1986, he was the first draft pick of the Boston Celtics. But only two days later, he died of a massive heart attack. Why? Because Len Bias had used cocaine.

Lucas, Johnson, Howe, Sanderson, Bias: these are just a few of the many athletes who have found themselves in trouble with drug use. But the use of drugs among athletes is not just a problem for a few. And it's not just a problem for the "stars," for the athletes with the big names and rich contracts. It's a problem for many amateur and college athletes, and more and more, it's a problem for young people in high school and even junior high school.

The use of drugs is a problem even for those athletes who never use them. For drugs spoil three main aspects of sports. First, drugs spoil the *fairness* of sports. By using steroids, Ben Johnson broke the rules of the Olympic games. He was caught and punished. But what about athletes who use drugs and don't get caught? Is it fair for drug-free athletes to lose to them?

Second, drugs spoil the *spirit* of sports. After all, sports are supposed to be athletic contests for healthy and talented players. But if a person is strong or fast because he took drugs like steroids, is he really a great athlete? Is this what sports are all about?

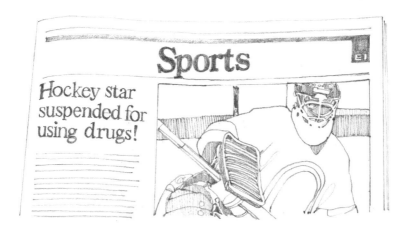

Third, drugs spoil the *image* of sports. Fans are beginning to think that *most* athletes take drugs. And even though this isn't true, it still hurts the players who are drug-free. Jack Lambert, a football Hall-of-Famer and a former defensive lineman for the Pittsburgh Steelers, says, "I run a football camp where I have to convince young kids that not all players use drugs. It's embarrassing." Randy White, formerly of the Dallas Cowboys, agrees: "I take good care of my body. But people just assume, 'Oh, he's a pro football player. He *must* do drugs.' That makes me mad."

The drugs that are most often used by athletes can be sorted into two main groups. The first group is called performance-enhancing drugs. The word "enhance" means "to make better." Some athletes think that these drugs will allow them to play better and harder and longer. Performance-enhancing drugs include amphetamines and anabolic steroids.

The second group of drugs used in the world of sports is called psychoactive drugs. These are drugs that people use to change the way they feel. Athletes use psychoactive drugs to wind down, to forget the many pressures they face, or just to get high. The most commonly used drugs in this group are alcohol and cocaine.

How widespread is the drug problem in sports? Let's look at some numbers.

• STEROIDS

Dr. Robert Voy, who is the chief medical officer of the U.S. Olympic Committee, estimates that more than half of the 9,000 athletes who competed at the 1988 Olympic games used steroids during training. Studies show that 85 percent of all professional football players have used steroids. Edwin Moses, a world champion track star, believes that "at least 50 percent" of the athletes in the high-performance sports (such as track and field, cycling, and rowing) use steroids.

One of the most recent surveys of teenage steroid use found that "large numbers of students in grades 7 through 12 use steroids" and that "the use of steroids among teens appears to be growing significantly." According to William Buckley, a health educator at the University of Pennsylvania, "Steroids are everywhere, whether a school is urban or rural, whether a user is an athlete or just wants to look good."

• COCAINE

Numerous studies show that at least 20 percent of professional baseball and football players have used cocaine. But some athletes who have been involved in cocaine use say the figure is much higher than that. Mike Strachan, a former football player with the New Orleans Saints who was convicted of selling cocaine to other players, says that between 40 and 60 percent of all National Football League (NFL) players have used cocaine. Carl Eller was an All-Pro defensive end with the Minnesota Vikings. He was also a cocaine addict. Eller says that between 40 and 50 percent of professional football players have used cocaine and that one out of every five players is a cocaine addict.

• ALCOHOL

Don Newcombe was a star pitcher with the Los Angeles Dodgers. He is also a recovering alcoholic.

Newcombe says that between 10 and 15 percent of all pro baseball players are alcoholics. Drug counselors think that the figure is even higher—that as many as 35 percent of the players are addicted to alcohol.

Today, alcohol use is the biggest drug problem in high-school and college sports. A recent study found that 90 percent of college athletes use alcohol regularly. A survey taken by the National Collegiate Athletic Association (NCAA) indicated that, nationwide, more than 30 percent of college athletes use alcohol during the playing season and more than 50 percent do so during the off-season. Other research reveals that the drinking problems of athletes frequently begin in high school. The state of Minnesota recently conducted a survey on the use of alcohol by high-school students. The results showed that as many as three out of every 10 high-school athletes use alcohol on a regular basis.

Of course, not all athletes use drugs. Many athletes are drug-free and are working to make the world of sports a drug-free one. And some of the athletes who have used drugs in the past are now working hard to help others take control of their lives again.

Carl Eller is one of them. Today, he works as a drug education consultant with the National Football League and heads a drug counseling center.

Derek Sanderson is one of them. Today, he heads a drug awareness program for young people.

And John Lucas is one of them.

John Lucas learned the hard way that drugs are tough to beat. But he is one of the lucky ones. John Lucas took control of his drug problem. He went into a long and difficult treatment program to recover from drug addiction. It was the hardest thing he ever did. Drugs are the toughest competitor he ever faced.

And, today, John Lucas works hard to help other athletes and young people get off and stay off drugs. He has helped other professional athletes through recovery programs. He leads an organization called STAND—"Students Taking Action, Not Drugs." Through STAND, Lucas helps young people who have used drugs move ahead with their lives. And he helps thousands of drug-free kids stay drug-free.

As John Lucas knows, the drug problem is one that starts early. It is one that many young people, whether or not they play sports, have to face:

> *"I've had an addictive personality ever since I was seven years old. I didn't do drugs then. But I wanted to be perfect. I was driven to do perfect work. Every coach wanted me on his team. Every time I scored a touchdown in football or made a free throw in basketball, I felt special. I felt perfect. My ego grew and grew. And drug addiction begins with ego. It begins with the feeling that you can beat anybody—or anything."*

For many young people, drugs may seem like an answer. They did for John Lucas:

"I was lonely as a kid. I had a lot of love from my family, but in my own mind I never measured up. And I never learned how to face my problems, how to cope. I turned to drugs as a solution to the problems I didn't know how to solve."

John Lucas knows now that drugs are a terrible "solution": "The government spends a lot of money trying to keep drugs from coming into the country," he says. "But the *problem* isn't coming in at the borders. The *problem* is here—guilt, shame, loneliness, anger, failure, lack of acceptance for who you are."

This is a book for young people. It is a book that will try to explain why talented athletes like Len Bias, John Lucas, Don Newcombe, and many others made the mistake of turning to drugs. In places, this book may make you sad. It may make you worry, too. It may make you wonder, "Could something like this happen to me?"

Athletes like John Lucas are working hard to give you the information you need so that drug problems *won't* happen to you. They hope that their stories will help you to stay healthy by saying "No" to drugs.

2

Why Athletes Take Drugs

"I decided I was going to take steroids to get big and strong and aggressive. I didn't care if I died, as long as I completed the season—just as long as I finished like a man."

—Tommy Chaikin, football player

"The pressure to take drugs is enormous. An athlete has to ask himself, 'Do I take drugs and win medals, or do I play fair and finish last?'"

—Augie Wolf, shot-putter

"You're in high school, and you want to be one of the guys. And the way you're one of the guys is to drink."

—Carl Eller, football player

"I was never one to look before I leaped. It's this simple: the drug was there, and I tried it. That sounds awfully stupid, and it was. I was a young man making a young man's bad mistake."

—Keith Hernandez, baseball player

This is how some athletes explain why they used drugs. There are other reasons, too. But all the reasons can be added together to form one big reason: athletes use drugs to try to solve or escape their problems.

In many ways, athletes are just like everyone else. They grow up in a world in which drugs are often used to solve problems. It's a world in which many people believe that drugs are the fastest way to solve a problem. Or the easiest way. Or even the only way. As Terry Taylor of the Seattle Seahawks says, "You grow up hearing commercials saying, 'You don't feel good? Take this drug. Can't sleep? Take that one.' It seems like there's an easy fix for everything."

Most of the problems that athletes face are not different from the problems that other people have to face. But because athletes are under such pressure to be "stars" or "heroes" or "the best," their problems may often seem to be too large to handle. Here are some of the reasons why athletes say they use drugs.

THE PRESSURE TO "FIT IN"

Everyone wants to be liked. It's true for athletes and nonathletes alike, for adults and young people. We especially want to be liked by our peers. Our peers are the people we spend time with, the people in our classes or on our sports teams. They're the people we want to be like.

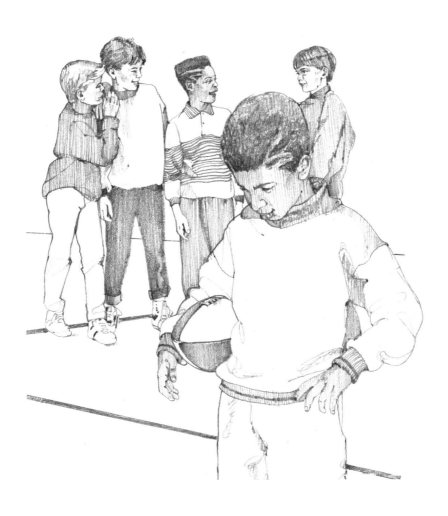

It's only natural to want to be liked by other people, but your peers can put pressure on you to be like them. They can put pressure on you to "fit in" or to be "part of the crowd." They can make you feel that you are not good enough as you are, that you should change to be more like them or that you should do what they do. We call this feeling peer pressure.

For many athletes, peer pressure means being tough. Derek Sanderson remembers that when he was growing up, he was always supposed to be tough:

> *"I was the toughest kid in the neighborhood. I wasn't afraid of physical pain. But I was afraid of emotional pain. So being tough meant that people would like me. And being tough meant that they'd respect me."*

And, for some, being tough means using drugs. "Drinking was just part of the 'good old boy' image," Sanderson says, "part of the 'Hey, I'm cool' image." Charles White, football's Heisman Trophy winner in 1979, agrees that peer pressure to use drugs is a major problem for athletes. "It was peer pressure that did it," he says. "I think that's really what got me started on using drugs. It was drinking beer after high-school games. You drank beer because you wanted to fit in with everybody."

For some athletes, peer pressure may mean the glamour of "life in the fast lane." It may mean moving from alcohol and marijuana to more expensive and glamorous drugs like cocaine. Former NBA All-Star Spencer Haywood says, "My wife and I became one of Hollywood's glamour couples. It just seemed like all of Los Angeles was getting high. You were embarrassed to admit you *didn't* use cocaine."

THE "UPS AND DOWNS" OF SPORTS

Perhaps baseball players know more about the ups and downs of sports than any other athletes do. Pitching stars can go into sudden slumps. Home-run heroes can fall into stretches of strikeouts. One day, the fans love a baseball player because he's on top. The next day, they call him a bum because his game is off. The changing attitude of the fans can make an athlete feel like a hero one day and a failure the next.

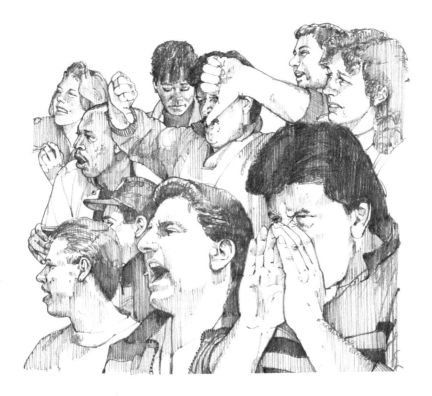

And, sooner or later, every athletic career comes to an end. Even those very few athletes whose dreams come true—who make it to the top—often find that they aren't on top for very long. An injury can suddenly end an athlete's career. Each year takes a little more edge off a player's game. And each year brings younger men and women, with stronger bodies and faster legs, to challenge the older players.

Most athletic careers are short ones to begin with. The average professional sports career lasts only four years. Sooner or later—usually sooner—the cheering stops, and the fans are rooting for someone else.

THE PRESSURE TO BE "THE BEST"

Many athletes are under constant pressure to win at all costs. They have to be "the best."

The pressure to win may mean putting on extra pounds of muscle to make the team. Some athletes use anabolic steroids as a chemical short cut to build up muscle tissue. The pressure to win may mean many hours of rigorous training. Steroids allow athletes to keep working out, even when they're tired and sore.

The pressure to win may mean playing with pain. Some athletes use amphetamines or other drugs so that they can play when they've been injured. Or the pressure to win may mean playing as aggressively, or even as violently, as possible. That's why some athletes use amphetamines to get "psyched" or "pumped up" before a game.

"No one realizes what goes on," says baseball player Willie Randolph about the pressure to be a great athlete. "It's pressure every day. It's a fishbowl. And not everybody's built to be so strong. Some can handle it, some can't. We're not superhuman."

The pressure to win comes from everyone.

• Parents put pressure on young athletes.

"Parents are pushing kids into athletics," says Dr. Wayne Moore of the University of Kansas. And they are pushing them at younger and younger ages. Even worse, some parents seem to accept the use of drugs as part of a young athlete's life. Over 50 percent of teenage steroid users say that their parents "probably know" they are using performance-enhancing drugs.

Many people think that parents who push their children to be stars on the athletic field do more harm than good. Young people can begin to think that winning is everything. They think that winning is a way to make sure they are loved, a way to be proud of themselves. These children learn a tough lesson at a very young age: if they lose, they think that they must be failures; they feel that they must be unworthy of love. Since most people do lose at some time, these young athletes can begin to see themselves as failures.

On the other hand, if they always seem to win, these young athletes may develop a feeling that they are special people—heroes who can do anything they want, champions who do not have to follow the rules. "Some players are spoiled little brats who have never grown up, who live in a sort of dream world," says football player Jack Lambert. "They're given special privileges and treated like royalty. They keep hearing about what great guys they are. The problem is that some of them start to believe it."

• Coaches put pressure on athletes.

Coaches want to win games just as much as athletes do. The coaches are under tremendous pressure to produce a winning team, and they can put that pressure on the athletes they lead. This might mean embarrassing or humiliating a player who has made a mistake or not played his best game. Former football player John Williams says, "If you make a mistake, the coach points it out to everyone. Meanwhile, inside, you feel like a volcano."

It might mean insisting that a player stay in the game even if he's injured. "I remember a coach saying to a player with a broken ankle, 'Okay, it's already broken. You can't break it again. Get out there and play,'" John Williams says. Basketball star Bill Walton certainly recalls the play-off game he played despite severe pain in his left foot. He was given an injection of a painkiller and sent back into the game. A few minutes later, he came out again—this time with a broken ankle, an injury that would hurt his basketball career for years.

The pressure might mean urging players to use performance-enhancing drugs or "looking the other way" when they do. Football player Tommy Chaikin recalls the pressure that led him to use steroids:

> *"I'd heard stories about the side effects of steroids. No way was I going to mess with something as risky as that. I was going to build myself up naturally. But the coaches wanted us to be as aggressive as possible, and it didn't matter where that aggression came from."*

This is how one sports doctor describes the effect of such pressure on young people:

> *"A coach will say to a kid, 'If you want to make first string, you've got to be 30 pounds heavier.' Well, the kid's been lifting weights like crazy to get his weight up to where it is now. All of a sudden, he's expected to gain 30 more pounds. Even though he may know that steroids will hurt him, he might be tempted to use them. Coaches have got to stop putting such killer risks on the shoulders of young people."*

- Athletes put pressure on themselves.

The greatest pressure that athletes face comes from inside themselves. They are driven to succeed. To many athletes, their whole identity as a person is wrapped up in the game they play. If they win the game, they feel like winners—not just as athletes but as people. If they lose, they feel that they are failures. Failures as athletes. Failures as people.

No one wants to fail. You want to do well on tomorrow's history test. Men and women in business want to do well in their jobs. The drive to do well is usually a good force in our lives. It makes us try hard and work hard. But sometimes the drive to do well can be too strong a force. It can make it impossible for us to accept ourselves for who we are, for what we have accomplished. It can make us feel like failures even when we have done our best, even when we have, in fact, accomplished a great deal.

Athletes, like everyone else, are under pressure to do well. But to many athletes, doing well means only one thing: it means winning. It means coming in first. If you take a history test, there are several grades you can get. An "A" is excellent. "B" means good. "C" is an average grade. A "D" means below average. And "F"—well, you know what "F" means. But to many athletes, there are only two grades: "A" and "F"; there is only winning and losing. There are no places in the

26

middle. It's win or lose. A "good" performance is just not good enough.

And, sometimes, success can be just as much of a problem as failure.

When Derek Sanderson signed a $2.3 million contract to play ice hockey with the Philadelphia Blazers, he was scared. "I was afraid that I wouldn't be able to perform like a star for the Blazers," he says. "I began to have thoughts like, 'Did I actually deserve all that money?'" Many other athletes who have also suffered from drug-related problems say that success, with the great expectations it brings, is the hardest thing of all to face.

There is one other reason why some athletes use drugs. They use drugs because they are addicted to them. Addiction is the constant need or craving for a drug. It means that drug use has changed the brain so much that it begins to need drugs. The brain of an addict needs drugs the way the brain of a healthy person needs natural and normal pleasures like food and sleep. That's why people who are addicted to drugs feel that they must have drugs. The only thing they think about is getting and using drugs. The only thing they care about is drugs.

The life of a professional athlete—a star—looks very good to us. It's a life filled with talent, fame, and money. But the life of a star isn't always as wonderful as we might think. It's also a life filled with tremendous pressures and fears. For some athletes, drugs are a way to cope with these pressures and fears.

And this life that seems filled with so much can also be a very empty one. It can be a very lonely life.

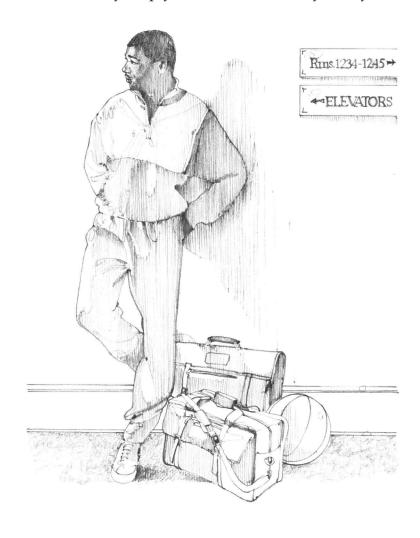

Rms. 1234-1245 →

← ELEVATORS

Because professional athletes have devoted so much of their time to their sport, many of them have few friends. They are "on the road" much of the season, playing games far away from family and loved ones. They are cheered on the field or the court, but when they come home, they are alone. For some athletes, drugs are a way to fill the emptiness.

There is no one reason why athletes use drugs. And there is no one answer to the problem of drugs and sports. When asked what he thought would help young people today, John Lucas had this to say:

"The simple ABCs of life are acceptance, believing, and caring. If you remember that, if you accept yourself for what you are, you'll be a winner. You'll be able to be proud of yourself for what you are inside, not just for what you do on the playing field."

Whether an athlete is young or old, whether an athlete uses performance-enhancing or psychoactive drugs, the drug problem is finally a problem of self-esteem. Self-esteem means believing in and accepting who you are. Self-esteem means being proud of what you've accomplished and confident about what you can do. That's why the solution to the drug problem is finally a matter of belief and confidence—of belief and confidence in what you can do without drugs.

It is a problem that John Lucas knows about.

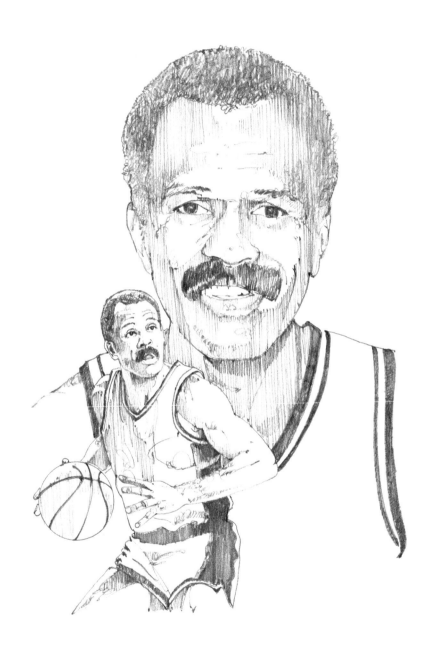

3

An Interview with John Lucas

John Lucas was born in 1953 and grew up in Durham, North Carolina. As a child, he excelled in both basketball and tennis. In college, at the University of Maryland, he was voted All-American in tennis once and in basketball three times.

His pro basketball career began with the Houston Rockets. Lucas also played for the Golden State Warriors, the Washington Bullets, the San Antonio Spurs, the Milwaukee Bucks, and the Seattle SuperSonics. He retired from pro basketball in 1990.

But John Lucas almost lost his basketball career to alcohol and cocaine. Three times he was suspended from professional basketball. Three times he tried to stop using drugs. In 1986, after a long and difficult treatment, he was successful.

Today, John Lucas lives in Houston, Texas, with his wife and two children.

Here, in his own words, is his story.

When and how did your problems with drugs begin?

Drug addiction for an athlete begins in elementary school. At least the kind of thinking that leads to drug addiction begins there. It did for me. I wanted to be perfect. And sports was a way to show that I was perfect. Most kids want to play sports because it's an ego thing—it's me against you, it's my team against your team, and we've got a winner. The game of life doesn't show any clear-cut winners, but sports does. And it's easy to feel like a winner in sports—work hard, compete, show no pain, and win at all costs. I wanted to be perfect, and that drive is characteristic of an addict.

How did wanting to be perfect lead to addiction?

Every coach wanted me on his team. Every time I scored a touchdown in football or made a free throw in basketball, I felt special. I felt perfect. My ego grew and grew. And drug addiction also begins with ego. It begins with a feeling that you can beat anybody—or anything.

Did you always win?

In the beginning, until I was 14, nobody ever beat me. So winning felt easy. But then people did start to beat me, and I felt like a failure. So I worked harder and harder and harder. I just couldn't accept losing. I just couldn't accept that there were some people who were bigger or stronger than I was. And I couldn't separate competing on the field from competing in the classroom or in everyday life. If I lost in a game, I felt lost as a person. I tried to be perfect in everything I did. And I kept coming up with failure.

But you were such a great athlete all the way through school. Didn't you win enough games to feel good about yourself?

No. I was never satisfied. I never stood back and said, "Good job, John." Every time I got to one goal, I was ready for the next one. I didn't have time to say, "Look at what I've accomplished." I was always pushing myself ahead to the next level of competition. In elementary school, I couldn't wait to get to junior high. In junior high, I couldn't wait to get to high school. In high school, I couldn't wait for college. And 701 colleges wanted me! Every coach wanted me to play for his team. But I couldn't be satisfied even then. I just couldn't wait to get to the NBA. I never felt good about where I was.

How would you help young athletes feel good about themselves?

I'd tell them to accept themselves. To understand that it's all a game and that it's just a sports uniform. What happens so often is that the athlete thinks that the uniform makes the person. But it doesn't. When I was in junior high, the principal would come on the microphone and say, "The Panthers are 15 and 0 for the season, and their leading scorer is John Lucas." You feel so special. And what happens is that every year your ego grows. And your acceptance of losing stops. The simple ABCs of life are acceptance, believing, and caring. If you remember that, if you can just accept yourself for what you are, you'll be a winner. You'll be able to be proud of yourself for what you are *inside*, not just for what you do on the playing field.

How can accepting yourself make you feel strong enough to say "No" to drugs?

Teaching a kid to stay off drugs has to begin with teaching a kid how to live—and how to cope with problems. Because what a kid has to accept today is easier than what he will have to accept tomorrow or next week. Problems get bigger the bigger you grow.

And when did your problems get too big to handle?

When I got to the pros. I was the first draft pick in 1976, and I went to the Houston Rockets. It was my last great goal. It was like the end of a life span for an athlete. I had started early, and I had trained hard. And now I was at the pros. But there was nothing bigger to go for. And now I was in a world where lots of people were better than I was. Because of the ego that I had developed as a kid, I had truly never believed in anything other than me. All I believed in was myself. So then, when I started finding out that there were people better than me, well, I just stopped believing in myself.

You don't *say* that to yourself. You don't say, "I don't believe in me." But you start looking around. And all that time, from the age of 7 to 14, I didn't. Because then I *was* the best. Then it was easy. I never looked around, and I never looked back. I just looked forward. What's the next level? What's the next level? Then, all of a sudden, somebody beats you. And you say, "Uh-oh. Who's coming up behind me? Who's next?" So you keep working for the next level of competition, the next level of accomplishment. But when you get to the pros, there *is* no other level. So then you start thinking, "Is this it? Am I a winner now?" I didn't *feel* like a winner. Because there were people better than me, I stopped believing in myself.

When did you turn to cocaine?

I'd used it once in college. But it came back when I was sent to California. The Rockets had to send someone, and California wanted either me or Moses Malone. And they chose to send me. It was the first time I had ever felt that somebody didn't want me on a team. And I freaked out. I had to move away from all my friends and family.

I got very, very lonely. I was away from home, wanting to make friends, wanting to be accepted. I remembered that back in college I had used cocaine when I was feeling lonely.

So I said to myself, "Aha! Drinks and drugs—they'll take the loneliness away."

But you were a star basketball player. Didn't you have friends on the team?

Most people don't understand that professional athletes are just like everyone else. You go to work with the other guys on the team. But after the game, or after the season, everyone splits. Everybody's got other interests—wives and family.

So I missed the friendships that college and high-school sports had given me. And I was lonely because I really didn't know how to make friends. All through school, I was working so hard to succeed at any cost that I never developed "kid" skills. I never learned how to play or relax. I never developed any interests to fill up my idle time.

And so the drugs filled the idle time for you?

Yes. Alcohol and cocaine became my new friends. They became my family. They became more important than my basketball.

They were more important than anything else in my life.

How did drugs affect your basketball skills?

I never played high, but I was playing very poorly. I wasn't sleeping or eating well, and I was losing weight. I was irritable. But I would never admit to myself that drugs were the problem. I blamed it on the coach. I even blamed it on the California weather. And then I started missing games. I felt I couldn't go to games because someone might see, might find out, that I was doing drugs.

When you saw that you weren't playing well, how did that fit in with your drive to be perfect?

It wasn't about being perfect anymore. All of my values—showing up for work and being responsible, being the kind of person I had been for years—went out the window. Drugs and alcohol were beginning to make me violate every value I ever had as a kid.

How did you finally stop using drugs?

Well, it was a long, long battle. California finally suspended me for missing games. I tried to stop drugs on my own. Then I went to Washington to play there. And the same pattern of drugs and alcohol started all over again. A reporter found out that I was an addict. He was going to print it in the paper. So I came out and admitted to the public that I had a drug problem.

The key is: I *admitted* the problem, but I didn't *accept* the problem. Not really. I tried to stop, but I didn't know how. I went into a drug treatment program that summer, but it didn't work. The following year, I was suspended after 35 games, this time from Washington. I went on to the San Antonio Spurs and then back to the Houston Rockets.

I felt good. I was home again. But in 1986, I had a positive urine test. Cocaine had finally got me. I was kicked off my team for the final time. My coach, Bill Fitch, said that I would never play basketball again. It was the worst moment in my life. I remember coming out of the Rockets' office with a suit and sunglasses on, trying not to be seen. And then my daughter went to school the next day, and all the kids said that her daddy was a druggie.

That year, the Rockets went to the NBA finals. Without me. They lost to the Boston Celtics. And the newspapers kept saying that all the Rockets needed to win was their point guard. The papers said the Rockets lost because of me.

As much as I didn't like what Bill Fitch did to me, I know today that he saved my life. Because I stayed sober—I stayed drug-free even with my team going to the finals without me, even with all of Houston blaming me for the Rockets' loss. I lived in this city during that. And I did it without drugs. Then I knew. I said, "Man, I can make it!"

Ten months later, after a lot of treatment and hard work, I was still drug-free. But it was the hardest thing I've ever done, getting off drugs. It's important for kids to know that.

In 1987, I went back to the NBA. I went to play for the Milwaukee Bucks. I never touched alcohol or cocaine again.

I had my best year ever as a pro that year. And I got over 2,000 letters from fans telling me about their kids' problems with drugs and asking me for advice. So I thought that I could help kids. And I could help other athletes, too.

And that's what I'm trying to do today.

I went through a terrible, terrible battle. Cocaine and alcohol will do everything people say they will do. They'll make you feel good when you're down. But they'll kill you.

And I'm lucky that I didn't get what I deserved. By doing cocaine, I deserved to be dead. What happened to Len Bias could just as easily have happened to me.

Does it embarrass you to be a recovering addict?

Not today. I accept who I am. And I'm not a phoney. I know who I am.

Finally, I understand that basketball and tennis are what I *do*. They're not who 1 *am*. For 32 years, I didn't know who I was. If someone had said, "Tell me who you are, John Lucas," I'd say, "I'm a basketball and tennis player."

And who are you today, John Lucas?

I'm a man. I'm a caring person. I'm a spiritual person. I'm a giving, loving, honest individual. I'm the best John Lucas I've ever been. And I know that life is a journey. There is only one highway in life, and you have to go the right way. You have to move forward and do the best you can. Because there are a whole lot of exits off that highway. And it's easy to make a terrible, terrible mistake. It's easy to get lost.

What would you say to the young people who read this book?

I would say, "Accept yourselves. And be proud of yourselves. Don't work so hard to succeed that you lose track of all the good things you've already done. And don't ever turn to drugs as a solution to your problems. I know what that's like."

4

The Performance Drugs

You know about the cartoon character Popeye. Whenever he's in trouble, whenever he needs extra strength to fight a bad guy or make a daring rescue, he rips open a can of spinach and eats it in one big gulp. Suddenly, like magic, his muscles bulge! He's the strongest man in the world!

Of course, you know it's just a cartoon. You know that spinach is good for you, but you also know that it can't make people as strong as Popeye's "magic" spinach. But throughout history, some athletes have turned to "magic" substances in the hope of finding extra help, extra strength, or extra confidence. They have turned to drugs to enhance athletic performance.

Over 2,000 years ago, at the very first Olympic games, Greek athletes ate special mushrooms before competing. These mushrooms, which contained drugs that change the way the brain works, helped the athletes to ignore their pain and their sore, tired muscles so that they could play longer and harder. In ancient Rome, chariot racers and gladiators also used drugs to mask the pain of their injuries. And other ancient athletes made a drink out of oil, rose petals, and crushed animal hooves. They drank this strange mixture because they believed it would increase their strength.

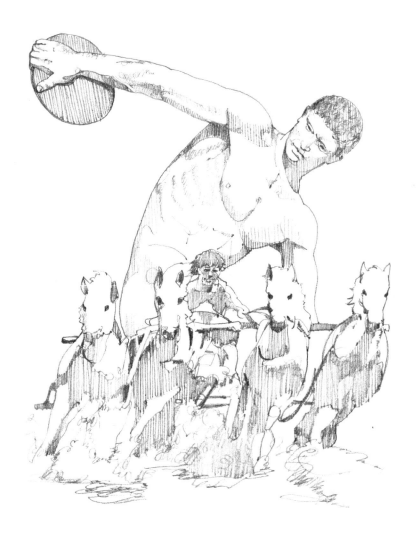

Even the slang word "dope" comes from the ancient world of sports. Before athletic competitions, the ancient Africans drank a mixture of alcohol and other substances that they called "dop." In the 1600s, people from Europe went to Africa to establish colonies there. They discovered the "magic" brew of dop and started using it, too. Over the years, the meaning of the word (now spelled "dope") changed. In the 1800s, it was defined as a combination of opium and other narcotic drugs given to racehorses to make them run faster. It was not long before human racers, and particularly marathon runners, were using a similar opium mixture before athletic contests. They hoped it would give them a "magical" speed and endurance.

In the late 1800s, some athletes began to use a drug called strychnine. Strychnine is a stimulant, a kind of drug that stimulates, or speeds up, the way the brain and body work. Strychnine stimulates the brain to make the body work harder and faster. But strychnine is also very poisonous. At the 1904 Olympic games, the winner of the marathon, American runner Tom Hicks, collapsed after crossing the finish line and fell into a coma. He had taken strychnine mixed with alcohol. Although Hicks did live, other athletes who used strychnine to enhance their sports performances were not that lucky. Today, we have found another use for strychnine: it is a powerful rat poison.

In the early 1900s, scientists would learn about other stimulant and body-building drugs. And, soon, other "magic" chemicals—drugs like amphetamines and anabolic steroids—entered the world of sports.

AMPHETAMINES

Modern athletes have turned in increasing numbers to stimulant drugs, especially the group of drugs called amphetamines. Often referred to as "pep pills," "uppers," or "speed," amphetamines came into widespread use in sports in the 1940s. Football players began to use them before games to get "pumped up." In the 1950s, the use of these stimulant drugs spread throughout the world of sports—to hockey, baseball, and bicycle racing, to the Olympics and college athletics. One study in 1958 estimated that almost 25 percent of college athletes had used amphetamines.

What kind of "magic" did these athletes find in stimulants? They found that amphetamines made them feel excited, tough, and "ready to go." Stimulant drugs also mask the sensation of pain, so athletes can compete even when injured.

But amphetamines can do a lot more than that. They can cause serious damage to the body, including stomach ulcers, weight loss, skin disorders, brain damage, and diseases of the lungs, liver, kidneys, and heart. Too strong a dose of amphetamines can even cause death from a sudden heart attack, from a stroke (a bursting of blood vessels in the brain), or from the failure of the lungs to keep breathing.

Amphetamines can also change the moods and emotions of the people who use them. The repeated use of amphetamines leads to nervousness, sleepless-ness, and depression. People who use amphetamines regularly become very irritable, easily upset, and suspicious of other people.

ANABOLIC STEROIDS

Anabolic steroids are a group of drugs used as a chemical short cut to a more muscular body. They are a synthetic, or laboratory-made, form of the natural male hormone testosterone. Like natural testosterone, anabolic steroids build up muscle tissue. The term "anabolic" means "tissue-building."

The natural male hormone testosterone produces the kinds of physical changes that turn a young boy into a man. When boys reach their teenage years, their bodies begin to change. They begin to develop the physical features of manhood. Their body hair be-comes thicker, their voices deepen, and their muscles develop. Because anabolic steroids are synthetic tes-tosterone, they produce the same kinds of physical changes, including bigger muscles, that the natural male hormone does.

By using anabolic steroids and working out, athletes can become bigger and stronger than they would be able to without drugs. Steroids also enable athletes to recover much more quickly from rigorous training sessions, so they can work out more often. Many athletes use steroids to build up muscles quickly. And some young people, both athletes and nonathletes, use them because they think a muscular body makes them look more attractive.

Anabolic steroids were first made in the 1930s. At that time, doctors thought they might prove to be useful medicines. They helped people who were suffering from conditions that made their bodies weak and frail. When they were given high-protein foods and steroids, these patients gained weight and strength.

Something else happened, too. Doctors noticed that steroids seemed to give their patients renewed energy and what can be called a "fighting spirit." This appeared to be good news. A tough, fighting spirit can give people the drive and will that are such an important part of recovery from serious illness.

The big muscles and fighting spirit that steroids gave to some medical patients made the drugs attractive to other people as well, including many athletes. In the 1950s, athletes in the Soviet Union and Eastern Europe started to use steroids. In 1954, an American sports doctor, John B. Ziegler, went to Europe as the physician for an American weightlifting team. There he found out about the use of anabolic steroids from a Soviet team doctor. Ziegler felt that the drugs gave the Soviets an unfair advantage. He thought that all athletes should benefit from these "wonder drugs." So Ziegler worked with a U.S. drug company to create anabolic steroids for American athletes—and he gave them to the members of his weightlifting team.

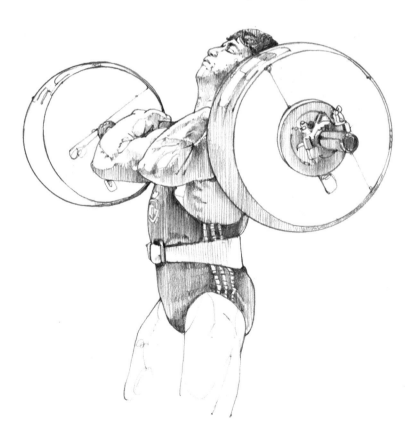

Ziegler thought that steroids were safe drugs. He tried them himself. He gave them to his weight lifters in small doses, and he checked the athletes carefully for side effects. The steroids enabled his athletes to train much harder and to lift much heavier weights. The American weight lifters were delighted with how these new drugs worked. They started to take more and more of them without Ziegler's approval. "They were eating them like candy," Ziegler later reported.

The word about these so-called "wonder drugs" quickly spread. Soon both male and female athletes in many sports—from football to swimming, from basketball to track and field—were using them. In 1988, the widespread use of steroids among athletes became very well known. That was the year that Ben Johnson, the Canadian track champion, was disqualified from the Olympic games and stripped of his gold medal after he tested positive for steroid use. But despite the widespread attention that Johnson's story brought to the steroid problem, athletes continue to rely on this chemical short cut.

Perhaps most alarming is the increasing use of steroids among young people. Today, one in every 15 male high-school seniors—over 500,000 teenagers—has used steroids. And according to two recent reports from the U.S. Department of Health and Human Services, "the use of these drugs among teens appears to be growing significantly." The studies found that the average age at which students start taking the drugs is 16 and that some begin as early as age 13.

What kinds of young people are using steroids? According to Robert Morris, executive director of the National High School Athletic Coaches Association, "These are motivated kids—kids who want to be better, stronger, faster. They want to achieve, and they see this as a short cut." Health and Human Services Deputy Inspector General Michael F. Mangano adds, "The scary thing is that kids do it for what society views as positive values: winning and success."

Also scary is the report's conclusion that many teachers, high-school coaches, and even parents are encouraging the use of anabolic steroids. Health and Human Services Secretary Louis W. Sullivan calls the findings disturbing: "I am very concerned," he writes, "that some adults who are charged with our young people's welfare might be accepting or even approving the use of these dangerous drugs."

Spinach may not give you the extra strength it gives to Popeye, but it won't hurt you to eat it. (In fact, as you have probably heard a hundred times, it really is good for you.) But steroids *will* hurt you.

Anabolic steroids are a form of testosterone, the body's natural male hormone. The flow of natural testosterone is controlled by the brain, which makes just the right amount of testosterone at just the right time. But using anabolic steroids upsets the natural balance of the body's hormones. It produces changes that are out of control. Steroid users often develop thick, shaggy hair growth on their arms and backs. Many athletes who use steroids report very heavy cases of acne, or pimples. And some go bald.

But these are only a few of the physical changes steroids cause, and they are not the most dangerous ones. Here are some of the more serious changes:

• Steroids can stop the body from growing.

Teenagers who take steroids often find out too late that these "wonder drugs" have actually stunted their growth. This happens because steroids cause the bones to stop growing normally. And even if the use of steroids is stopped, the bones will not grow any further. Dr. Robert Cantu, a leading expert in sports medicine, says, "A teenage boy who uses steroids is making a bad trade. He's going to gain some body bulk, to be sure. But he's going to pay for that bulk by throwing away inches and inches of height."

• Steroids can shrink the testicles.

When the body receives anabolic steroids, it stops producing real testosterone on its own. The body is "fooled" into thinking that it has a sufficient supply of the natural male hormone. Since the testicles, the male sex glands, are no longer producing testosterone, they grow inactive and shrink. This can be a permanent condition: the testicles may never look normal again. Using steroids can also interfere with the ability of the testicles to produce sperm, or reproductive, cells. Some young boys who use steroids may never be able to father children.

• Steroids can cause men to lose the signs of maleness.

The body of a man or a boy makes female hormones as well as male hormones. By using steroids, a man causes his body to stop producing testosterone. However, his body will continue to make the female hormones. This can cause a male steroid user to lose some of the physical signs of his maleness. It can even lead to an enlargement of the breasts. Doctors have reported performing mastectomies, or breast removal operations, on young men who used steroids.

• Steroids can create special problems for women.

Just as the body of a boy or a man makes female hormones, so a woman's body makes a small amount of testosterone. But when a woman uses steroids, her body's natural balance of male and female hormones is upset. A woman who uses steroids is giving her body too much testosterone, and she may begin to develop the physical signs of maleness. Her body begins to look more and more like the body of a man.

Many women who use anabolic steroids develop excessive facial and body hair. Their breasts get smaller, and their voices deepen. They may begin to go bald. The use of steroids can also interfere with the normal functioning of the woman's reproductive system, and women who use steroids may lose the ability to have babies. These changes are often permanent.

• Steroids can damage the body's tendons.

Tendons are the tough, elastic tissues that connect muscles to bones. The use of steroids can cause the tendons to become brittle and break. The tendons are unable to stretch and bend as they are supposed to when the muscles move. Some weight lifters who use steroids have suffered from broken tendons. One power lifter describes what that felt like:

"I felt something pop inside my arm. It felt like a rubber band snapping. I heard a sound like a big rip. My tendon had snapped. My bicep just bunched all up. It rolled up my arm, like a window shade."

• Steroids can damage the heart, liver, and kidneys.

Heart disease is the leading cause of early death among steroid users. And the victims are often very young. The story of one high-school football player who took steroids is typical. He took steroids to "bulk up" for the football season. Three days after his "big game," in which he led his team to a 21-6 victory, he had a heart attack and died. The doctors said his heart was damaged by steroids. He was only 17 years old. Steroids can also damage the veins and arteries that allow blood to circulate throughout the body.

Steroids can harm the liver and kidneys. At 26, Birgit Dressel was a world track star. Dressel was a champion in the heptathlon, a strenuous seven-part track and field event. She was training hard, hoping to win a gold medal in the 1988 Olympic games. But, in 1987, following a routine practice session, she felt stabbing pains in her back. She died later that night. Steroids had ruined her liver and kidneys.

And there are additional side effects to steroids. These drugs not only change the way the body works. They can change the way the brain works, too. They can change the way a person thinks, feels, and acts.

The fighting spirit that comes with steroid use often runs out of control, producing angry and violent outbursts. This violent behavior is so common among steroid users that it has been given its own name— "roid rage." Tommy Chaikin says:

"Images of violence used to fill my mind. I'd be driving along and find myself thinking about sick things like crushing people to death, tearing off their arms and legs. I'd be grinding my teeth and gripping the wheel so hard that my arms would hurt."

Steroids can cause other changes to the thoughts and emotions of the people who use them. They make some users feel very nervous or suspicious. A typical reaction is to think that everyone is "out to get me." Again, from Tommy Chaikin:

> "I was starting to battle anxiety attacks that I was sure were caused by steroids. I can't really describe an attack, except to say that it's like your mind is a car engine stuck in neutral with the gas pedal to the floor, just screaming. There's terror mixed in, and you think you're going to explode."

Steroids make others feel so strong and powerful that they think nothing can hurt them. Using steroids can make it very hard for a person to fall asleep and cause terrible nightmares once sleep finally comes. Some steroid users hear voices that don't exist. And many users become moody and depressed when they try to stop using steroids.

With all of these dangers to the body and mind, why do athletes continue to use steroids?

Some athletes refuse to believe that the drugs will hurt them. They fool themselves into believing that they'll be lucky. They think they'll be tougher than steroids. They think they can control steroids.

Other athletes believe that they'll be safe because they'll take steroids for just a short while—until they gain the weight they want or until they reach a certain level of weightlifting. But once a person starts to take steroids, it is very hard to stop. If he or she does stop, the muscles shrink back to their normal size. It seems like a cruel trick: a person's body may be permanently damaged, but the big muscles are just a temporary "benefit." Many steroid users say that they have tried to stop, but couldn't. They hate to lose those muscles.

And some athletes, driven to be the best at all costs, decide that the risks of using steroids are worth it. But, of course, they aren't.

OTHER DANGEROUS DRUGS

There are several less common drugs that some people have used to enhance athletic performance.

One of these new drugs is called human growth hormone (hGH). Human growth hormone is a natural chemical (a chemical the body makes) that stimulates and regulates body growth. Synthetic hGH is sometimes used as a medicine to help children who are not growing normally. It is also being used today by some athletes. Athletes have turned to human growth hormone because they believe that hGH can make them stronger. They have also turned to it because human growth hormone, unlike amphetamines and steroids, cannot be detected by drug tests.

They have turned to a drug that scientists know very little about. Scientists do not yet know whether hGH actually does make people stronger. And they do not know all of the side effects that the drug may have on the body. However, many studies show that hGH can cause acromegaly, a painful condition that causes the bones in the face to grow out of shape.

There are other, less commonly used drugs that are part of the world of sports. A variety of drugs, including narcotics (or opiates) such as morphine, are used to treat pain. Some athletes use depressants or a group of drugs called beta-blockers to help control the pressure of athletic performance. Other athletes use diuretics, a group of drugs that flush out liquids from the body, to lose weight before important events or to flush out any trace of drugs before they are tested.

These are some of the drugs used by athletes who think they need a chemical short cut to enhance their strength, speed, or stamina. And in the years ahead, developments in science and medicine will lead to the discovery of new performance-enhancing drugs. But those athletes who do use such drugs to enhance their natural abilities may be kidding themselves. Recent studies suggest that the use of these drugs, including amphetamines and steroids, may, in fact, do very little to enhance a person's athletic performance. They are certain, however, to have unintended, unwanted, and unhealthy side effects that may do serious damage to the body and brain.

5

The Psychoactive Drugs

The same pressures that lead some athletes to use performance-enhancing drugs can also lead to the use of other drugs. The pressure to fit in, the pressure to win, the pressure of the "ups and downs" of sports, and the pressures of failure and success—these are the kinds of pressures that lead many athletes to want to escape, to hide for a moment from the world that Willie Randolph calls the "fishbowl" of sports.

It's only natural to want to escape from the pressures of our lives. It's only normal to look for an easy solution to our problems.

But too often today, for both athletes and nonathletes, the easy answer is one that offers no escape from life's pressures and no solution to life's problems. It's an answer that only makes things worse. Too often, the easy answer is drugs.

Several kinds of drugs that people use to change the way they feel are known as psychoactive drugs. A psychoactive drug is a substance that changes the way the brain works. It changes the way people think, feel, and behave. The two psychoactive drugs most commonly used by athletes today are alcohol and cocaine (and crack, a form of cocaine). Of course, these drugs are not just problems for the world of sports.

- There are more than 10 million alcoholics in the United States. Each year, more than 100,000 people die from diseases due to alcohol, and over 500,000 people have to enter drug treatment programs for alcoholism. Today, more than 5 million teenagers have serious drinking problems. More than half of them started using alcohol before the tenth grade.

- Over 21 million people in the United States have used cocaine. In 1990, over 8 million people used the drug, and the number of people addicted to cocaine is increasing. In the last few years, crack, a form of cocaine that is made to be smoked, has spread to every city and town. And, like alcohol, cocaine is a major problem for young people. One in every 10 teenagers tries cocaine. The average age of a crack user is only 17 years old.

But the use of psychoactive drugs by athletes is a special problem. It's a special problem because many athletes do live in a fishbowl. When they are caught using drugs, it's front-page news. It's a special problem because athletes, whether they like it or not, serve as role models for us, especially for young people. We want to look up to athletes, to admire them. We wish we could be more like them. And we want them to be perfect. We don't want our sports heroes to have the same problems that other people have.

But they do. And like other people, many athletes try to run away from their problems by using drugs.

Different psychoactive drugs do different things to the brain. It's important to know these differences.

- Alcohol is a kind of drug called a depressant. It depresses, or slows down, the messages to and from the brain that control our senses, movements, thoughts, and emotions.

- Cocaine is a kind of drug called a stimulant. It stimulates, or speeds up, the messages to and from the brain that control our senses, movements, thoughts, and emotions.

But it is also important to understand one thing, perhaps the most important thing, that is the same for both these drugs. Both alcohol and cocaine are highly addictive drugs. The repeated use of these drugs leads to such serious changes in the way the brain works that it can become very hard for people to stop using them—even when they want to. Using these drugs can lead to the sickness of drug addiction.

Psychoactive drugs like alcohol and cocaine (or crack) change the way the brain sends the messages that control our thoughts and emotions. The repeated use of these drugs can permanently upset the balance of important chemicals within the brain. That's why using these drugs can cause important changes in the way the brain works.

- Both drugs lead to tolerance, which means that users need more and more of the drug to get the same effects. What happens is that the nerve cells of the brain get used to the effects of the drug, so the same dose of the drug no longer speeds up or slows down the brain as much as it used to.

- Both drugs lead to dependence, which means that users need the drug to feel normal. When the drug is taken away, users suffer from the pains of drug withdrawal. In other words, without the drug, they feel very sick.

Addiction means that drug users need more and more drugs just *not* to feel sick. It means that drug addicts are driven by their own brains to use drugs. It also means that drug use becomes the most important thing in a person's life. Nothing else—not family and friends, not school or work—is as important to them as drugs.

Drug addiction is a sickness, and drug addicts need help. It is very hard for addicts to stop using drugs. They need medical treatment and drug counseling. But many people who are addicted to drugs deny that they even have a drug problem. They deny it to others. And they deny it to themselves.

Addicts can get help, and they can get better. But, first, they need to admit that a drug problem exists. And even more, they have to *accept* that a drug problem exists. Before anyone can help them, drug addicts have to accept that they need help.

Let's look at how dangerous drugs can be.

• ALCOHOL

When he was eight years old, Derek Sanderson knew exactly who he was. He was a great hockey player. He knew it because his father, who was also his coach, told him so. But he knew it inside himself, too. He knew he had the talent. It was easy to see. He knew he had the strength. And maybe most important of all, Derek knew he had the right attitude—tough enough to practice and play hard, and fearless enough to risk getting hurt.

Hockey is a rough game. The first time that Derek got hit, he felt shock and pain. Blood was streaming down his face. It was all over his sweater. He skated out of the game. "Dad, I'm cut!" he moaned.

"Yes, I know," his father answered. "But you can't quit now. There's 20 minutes left in the game."

So Derek skated back into the game. "Look at Derek," he heard the other kids say. "He's still going to play. He's really tough."

"Do you know who you are, Derek?" he said to himself. "You're a great hockey player!"

Derek Sanderson was a tough kid and a tough player. And as he grew up, his talents and his toughness grew, too. In 1968, in his first season with the Boston Bruins, he was voted National Hockey League Rookie of the Year. He went on to help the Bruins win two Stanley Cup championships in 1970 and 1972. Then he signed a $2.3-million contract with a new team, the Philadelphia Blazers of the World Hockey Association. It was a lot of money; it was a fantastic deal. Derek Sanderson was on top of the world.

Now Derek Sanderson really had it all—he had talent, fame, and money. He seemed to have everything. But he had something else, too—something that made him slide off the top of the world. Derek Sanderson had a drug problem. He was addicted to alcohol and other drugs.

His career disappeared. His fame disappeared. And all the money disappeared, too. It all went for drugs. One day, Derek Sanderson, the great hockey star, was huddled under a bridge in a city park. He had lost it all. But at that moment, he wasn't thinking about hockey. He was thinking about where he could find the money to buy himself a drink.

He saw another man huddled nearby, drinking out of a bottle. He asked the man to give him a drink, too. But the man said, "No." Derek was angry. How could this man turn down Derek Sanderson, the great hockey player?

"Do you know who I am?" he shouted at the man.

"Yes," said the man. "You're a drunk."

Sometimes, it must seem that alcohol and sports just go together. Beer and other alcoholic drinks are sold at many athletic events. Advertisements and commercials for alcoholic products often feature athletes drinking together. Companies that make beer and other drinks sponsor many athletic competitions, from tennis tournaments to speedboat races. Even post-game victory parties show us the winning athletes celebrating with champagne.

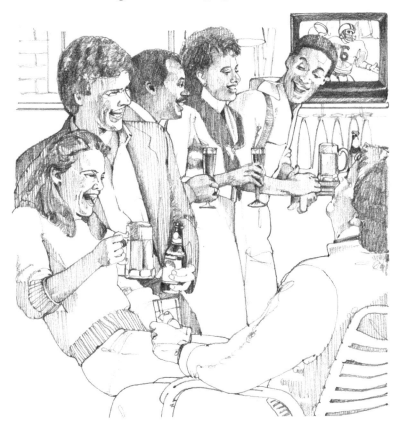

What is this drug that seems so much a part of sports, and what does it do?

Alcohol enters the bloodstream through the stomach and intestines and, because it does not have to be digested, is carried quickly to the brain. As a depressant, alcohol disrupts the messages traveling to and from the brain that control our senses and movements, our thoughts and emotions. Alcohol makes it hard to see and hear clearly. It can make it hard to walk and even to stand up. Alcohol disrupts the messages that direct our thoughts, making it hard to concentrate and to remember things. And it disrupts the messages that control our emotions, making people happy or sad, angry or depressed, for no reason.

The repeated use of alcoholic products can permanently damage the body. It can cause serious harm to the liver, kidneys, stomach, brain, and heart. It can lead to some kinds of cancer. And if pregnant women use alcohol, it can cause health problems for their unborn children.

Alcohol is often called a "gateway drug." This means that alcohol may lead to the use of other drugs. Many athletes with drug problems report that alcohol is the drug they first used. John Lucas began to drink when he was a teenager. In high school, Carl Eller drank to be "one of the guys." One recent survey shows that three out of every 10 high-school athletes use alcohol on a regular basis.

And professional athletes are part of the reason why young people use alcohol. Many people feel that the world of sports needs to take a firmer stand on alcohol. They think that alcohol should be taken out of the locker rooms and that athletes should not make advertisements for alcoholic products. Young people naturally look up to famous athletes. When athletes appear in beer commercials, does this make drinking beer look like something that kids should try, too?

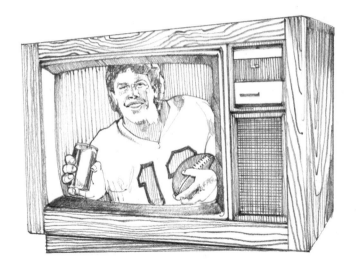

Some athletes who have had drug problems think it does. "When someone tells kids, 'Try this, you'll feel great, it can't hurt,' they may well go ahead and try it," says Derek Sanderson. "But they might not try it if someone would tell them the truth: you try it and you get hurt—*bad*."

Of course, alcohol is dangerous to use even if it doesn't "open the gate" to further drug use. Baseball player Bob Welch, a talented pitcher, knows just how dangerous it can be. Welch is a recovering alcoholic who goes to high schools to caution young athletes about the dangers of alcohol. He says:

"I was in high school just a few years ago. If some doctor or teacher had said to us, 'Alcohol is dangerous,' we would have laughed in his face. But if a ball player or somebody closer to my age had warned me, maybe I would have listened. I hope young people listen to me now."

Chris Mullin, a star performer on the basketball court, knows how dangerous alcohol can be. Mullin was an All-American in college, a member of the U.S. Olympic team, and the first-round draft pick of the Golden State Warriors. But his drinking nearly ruined a promising career. "It got to the point where it wasn't that I wanted alcohol," he says, "but that I *needed* it."

Professional golfer Sally Quinlan also knows how dangerous alcohol can be. "I should have realized in college that something was wrong," she now admits. "I'd go to my classes with the worst hangovers. I'd miss golf because of it. But I always thought an alcoholic was an old man in a raincoat in the gutter. I figured I was too young, too athletic, too smart to be an alcoholic."

• COCAINE

According to Dr. Mark S. Gold, the founder of a national drug hotline, it is the most popular drug in the world of sports.

According to a New York newspaper, 50 percent of professional football players use it.

The drug is cocaine.

What is cocaine, and what does it do?

Cocaine is a powerful stimulant that comes from the leaves of the South American coca plant. Cocaine is known by many street names, including "coke," "snow," "blow," and "flake." A white mixture that looks like powdered sugar or baby powder, cocaine may be sniffed through the nose or injected directly into the bloodstream with a hypodermic needle. One very addictive form of cocaine, called crack, is made to be smoked. It comes in small, hard chips that look like little slivers of soap.

Like other stimulants, cocaine speeds up the way the brain and the body work. It makes the heart and lungs work faster. Cocaine produces a strong sense of pleasure and energy, but the cocaine high lasts only about 20 minutes. It is followed by a "crash," a sick feeling that drug users often get when the effects of a stimulant drug wear off. A cocaine crash can make users feel nervous, depressed, angry, tired, and upset. That's why cocaine users often want to use the drug again. They want to feel the pleasurable sensations of the cocaine high, and they want to avoid or at least postpone the painful feelings of the cocaine crash.

That's why cocaine is so highly addictive. That's why many people who study the effects of drugs say it is easier to get hooked on cocaine than on any other drug. That's why two out of every three callers to the national 800-COCAINE hotline say that they are unable to stop using coke even though, according to hotline founder Mark Gold, "they know it is destroying their lives."

Cocaine damages the body. It causes headaches, vomiting, nosebleeds, sore throats, coughing, sinus problems, and muscle pains. Because it disrupts the regular pumping of the heart, cocaine can lead to sudden heart attacks. It can also permanently damage the brain and the lungs.

Cocaine also changes the way people think and act. It can cause users to get edgy, easily upset, and highly suspicious of other people. It may make some users so depressed that they begin to think about killing themselves. Cocaine users may also suffer from hallucinations, which are distortions of normal sights and sounds. But more than anything, cocaine addicts feel a craving for more and more cocaine.

Unlike alcohol, cocaine is not legal for adults to use. You won't see it advertised on television or hear jingles for cocaine on the radio. You won't see athletes endorsing a cocaine product or see cocaine producers sponsoring an athletic competition. But most professional athletes agree that it's not hard to get cocaine.

The New York Mets pitching ace Dwight Gooden describes how some athletes get started on cocaine:

> *"You're at a party, and someone says, 'Hey, have some of this.' First it's free, but then it costs. You go through a whole heap of money. Looking back, you think you'd have been better off just ripping the money up and throwing it into the ocean. The lesson is that there's no free ride. You start with drugs, and you're going to pay and pay and pay."*

And the cost of using cocaine can be far greater than money.

John Drew became a cocaine addict while he was playing basketball with the Atlanta Hawks. It ruined his career and put him into prison. He warns:

> *"There are three things that can happen to you when you get hooked on coke. One is to go to jail. Another is to get help. The third is death. It will kill you. Believe me, cocaine will kill you dead."*

That's what cocaine did to Len Bias. Many people thought Len Bias was the best college basketball player in the country. But cocaine killed him at the age of 22, just two days after he was drafted by the Boston Celtics.

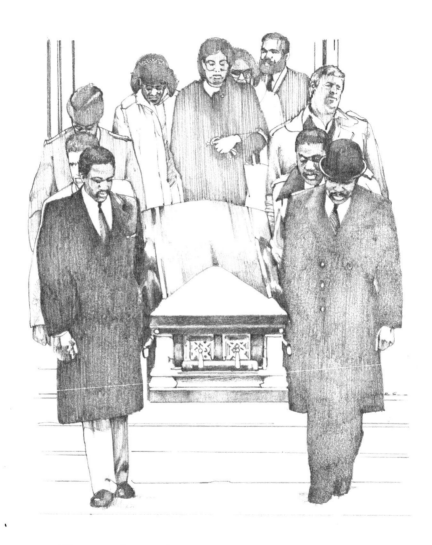

That's what it did to Don Rogers, a safety for the Cleveland Browns. The day before he was to be married, he died of a heart attack brought on by cocaine. He was 23 years old.

Cocaine has hurt many others.

It has hurt football players like Dexter Manley, Thomas "Hollywood" Henderson, Larry Bethea, Pete Johnson, Carl Eller, Tony Peters, and Ross Browner.

It has hurt baseball players like Juan Bonilla and Dwight Gooden.

It has hurt basketball players like John Drew, Roy Tarpley, David Thompson, and John Lucas.

It has hurt hockey players like Grant Fuhr and Derek Sanderson.

There are hundreds of professional and amateur athletes whose careers have been hurt by cocaine.

With so much at risk, why would athletes want to try psychoactive drugs? What do athletes who start to use these drugs say to themselves?

• They may say, *"I'll just try it to see what it feels like. I won't get addicted to drugs."*

That's what Juan Bonilla, second baseman for the San Diego Padres, said. Today, Bonilla is a recovering cocaine addict. He remembers how he felt when he began to use drugs:

> *"You say to yourself, 'Don't worry—I can do it today and quit tomorrow.' That's a mistake. We're not talking about an error you can make up for with a late-inning, game-winning hit. We're talking about life and death."*

71

- They may say, *"I'm tough and talented. I won't get hurt by drugs."*

That's what Gary McLain, a star basketball player at Villanova University, said. "Fear was the one thing I lacked," McLain remembers. "Back then, I always thought that I was in control of everything. I thought I could handle cocaine."

John Lucas knows the same feeling. "It's a hard concept for an athlete to believe," he says, "the idea that I can play great basketball in front of over 20,000 people and a little white powder is going to beat me."

- They may say, *"I'm not addicted. I may have a drug problem, but I can handle it."*

It's hard for people to admit that they need help. It's especially hard for a person who's been trained to be tough. That's why it's easy for an athlete to deny, or refuse to admit and accept, that he or she has a drug problem. John Lucas says:

> *"Your brain is always trying to trick you, telling you that you don't have a problem. But you do. There's no way to get around it and no way to ignore it. As an athlete, I'd always been taught to try to win at any cost. But in order to beat this disease, I finally realized I had to surrender to it. I had to admit that it had beaten me. I had to get help."*

- They may say, *"Everyone in sports is using drugs."*

It may seem that way, but it certainly isn't true. The world of sports does, in fact, have a serious drug problem. But there are many athletes who never use drugs. And there is good reason to believe that, in the future, an increasing number of athletes will be drug-free. As we shall see in the next chapter, the world of sports is taking a tough stand on drug use, and more and more athletes are leading the fight against drugs.

- They may say, *"So what if I get addicted? I can stop later. If other athletes beat addiction, so can I."*

Athletes who have suffered from drug addiction would agree on one important thing: no one can beat drug addiction. Spencer Haywood says:

> *"Somebody told me that by telling my story I was letting people know it's okay to do drugs, because you can eventually clean yourself up and everything's cool. Well, it's never cool. I can never get back what I threw away. I can never repair the damage drugs did to my personal life."*

But no matter what they say to themselves, athletes who use drugs are making a mistake—a mistake that one day could cost them their careers, a mistake that one day could cost them their lives.

6

Where Do We Go from Here?

The world of sports has a drug problem. And most people agree that there is no easy answer, no one simple way to solve the problem. But many amateur sports organizations, like the National Collegiate Athletic Association (NCAA) and the International Olympic Committee (IOC), and professional organizations such as the National Football League and the National Basketball Association are trying hard to find as many ways as possible to help rid the world of sports of the drug problem.

Drug testing is one way. If a player has used such drugs as steroids, amphetamines, cocaine, or alcohol, traces of the drugs will show up in the player's urine. For more than 25 years, urine tests have been used to detect drugs in the bodies of athletes. Over the years, the tests have become more and more accurate. Now, even the tiniest traces of foreign substances can be detected. In fact, the drug-testing lab at the University of California at Los Angeles boasts that its testing procedures are so accurate and foolproof that they could tell if a spoonful of sugar had been dumped into an Olympic-sized swimming pool!

But with drug testing have come other concerns. Some people feel that a player should not be forced to take a urine test. They feel that such testing violates the player's legal right to privacy. Other people worry that the tests can make mistakes—they may show a positive result for illegal drugs even if the player has taken only a legal painkilling drug.

And many people who are "for" drug tests don't agree with the way most tests have been conducted. Until recently, most tests were scheduled, so players knew when their urine would be tested. Most tests were held just before a game or race. This meant that players could use drugs through their training period and then stop a few days before the test. That way, traces wouldn't show up in their urine. Or they could take other drugs, such as diuretics, to try to flush all traces of drugs out of their systems.

Recently, The Athletics Congress (TAC) started a tough drug-testing program for all amateur track and field athletes. They ruled that an athlete who's ranked within the top 15 in an event could be required to provide a urine sample at any time during the year. The athletes would be notified only 36 hours before the test. And at their annual convention in January 1990,

NCAA officials voted to establish a program of year-round random testing. These sports groups think that if players don't know when the tests will be held, they will have a far harder time "hiding" their drug use—during training *and* competition. NCAA Executive Director Dick Schultz doesn't think that random drug testing alone can solve the problem, but Schultz and other athletic officials see the new drug-testing policy as a "good first step."

Random drug testing is also beginning to be used in high-school athletic programs. At the Homewood-Flossmoor High School in Chicago, every student in interscholastic sports is participating in a testing program. Visiting nurses pick a sample group of student athletes for urine tests. If a student tests positive for drugs, he or she must take a second test. If the second test is positive, the student must enter a counseling and treatment program.

Several athletic organizations have attempted to use random drug testing to insure that all competitors are drug-free. The National Football League is now using random drug tests as a standard part of pre-season camp to make sure that players arrive for the season drug-free. And all over the country, weight-lifting groups such as the American Drug-Free Power-lifting Association are making their competitors undergo random tests and sign a contract that states that they are drug-free.

Another way that sports organizations have tried to attack the drug problem is to punish drug-using athletes by banning them from games, by suspending them from their teams, or by making them pay fines. And several athletes who have been caught using or selling illegal drugs have gone to prison.

But one group of people who have a role in the drug problem continues to be free of any punishment. Many athletes say that their coaches knew about the use of steroids by team members. Other athletes have even reported that amphetamines and steroids were handed out in the locker room. When Ben Johnson was caught using steroids, his coach and team doctor admitted that they had urged him to use the drugs—yet they suffered no punishment.

Today, many athletes and sports officials feel that coaches and doctors who advise or encourage their players to use drugs should be punished and perhaps banned from the world of sports. Edwin Moses is an athlete who feels that way. He is probably the greatest 400-meter hurdler of all time. During one nine-year period, he won 122 races in a row. Moses won gold medals at the 1976 and the 1984 Olympics, a bronze medal in 1988, and now plans to compete in the 1992 Olympics, too. Moses is also a leader in the drug-free sports movement. He has recently taken a full year off from training to help the U.S. Olympic Committee begin a program to stop drug use by athletes. He has also volunteered to help other sports organizations set up drug education, research, testing, and counseling programs.

Edwin Moses proposes two simple steps to attack the drug problem in sports: (1) random testing for all athletes during training periods, and (2) punishment of all coaches, trainers, and managers who assist or encourage an athlete to take drugs. He says:

"We'll make no progress if we snip off the last link in the chain, such as the runner Ben Johnson, and allow the guilty members of his support crew to move on to the next athlete."

The National Collegiate Athletic Association has tried to set up rules to protect college athletes, and college sports in general, from the problems of drug abuse. But many people feel that their rules are either not strong enough or not enforced carefully enough. For example, the NCAA rules state that to compete in college sports, a player must be enrolled as a student. But in many cases, the specific rules about attending classes and getting good grades are left to individual colleges to set. Some colleges demand that their athletes follow the same rules imposed on other students. But, sadly, many colleges do not.

And at many schools, athletes are not encouraged to mix with nonathletes or even to participate in other school activities. They often live together in one dorm, away from other students, and are not supervised by anyone except members of the athletic coaching staff. Statistics and case studies show that many college athletes end up leaving college without earning enough credits to graduate. In fact, some are not even able to read or write.

Many teachers and counselors feel that without academic and personal guidance during their college years, amateur athletes are more prone to problems than other students are. Further, counselors think that the athletes' lack of a meaningful education and interests other than sports often prevents them from being able to deal with their problems effectively. They may turn, as many have turned, to an escape from those problems. They may turn to drugs.

Some professional sports leagues are now helping drug-using players by supporting the treatment programs of local clinics or hospitals. Some teams are establishing their own programs to help their players get off, and stay off, drugs. Former NFL coach Sam Rutigliano set up a group called "The Inner Circle," where players met once a week for group counseling and support.

Other NFL teams have benefited from the work of Carl Eller, a recovering cocaine addict. Once an All-Pro lineman with the Minnesota Vikings, Eller works today as a consultant to the NFL drug prevention and education programs. Eller has also set up a private drug counseling and treatment center in Minneapolis, Minnesota, called Triumph Life. He is credited with helping many drug-addicted athletes.

Eller is not the only recovering drug addict and former professional athlete who is working hard to help other players with drug problems. Several athletes who know firsthand how damaging drugs can be are working today to help other people avoid the problems of drug use. And their work is aimed not just at athletes. They hope to help *all* young people find the self-confidence to say "No" to drugs.

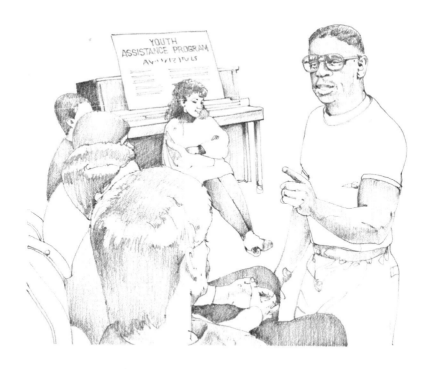

In addition to his Triumph Life Center, Carl Eller also runs a group known as the United States Athletes Association. Through this agency, kids get together to play sports and talk. Eller helps young people to become leaders within the group. The student leaders, he says, become models to other students. They show the other students how much can be accomplished by being healthy and drug-free.

Derek Sanderson goes to high schools and junior high schools throughout the New England area, sharing his own story with young people. Once one of the toughest men on a hockey rink, Sanderson is now one of the toughest fighters against drug use. During his talks at schools, he asks all teachers to leave the room. He wants to make kids as comfortable as possible. He wants them to talk openly about the pressures and problems in their lives.

In Detroit, Spencer Haywood started the Spencer Haywood Foundation. Through it, more than 3,000 young people in the city of Detroit get to go to basketball camp during the summer. Haywood, one of the game's great centers, now teaches young people how to play the game. He also works hard to be someone they can talk to about their problems and worries. He feels that if people solve their "living" problems, perhaps they won't feel the need to look to drugs as some kind of solution or escape.

John Lucas agrees with that approach to the drug problem. He believes that the best way to try to solve the drug problem is to help people find better solutions to the problems that might lead them to drugs.

Lucas has put a drug counselor in every city that has an NBA team so that pro basketball players with drug problems can turn to someone for help. He has established the John Lucas New Spirit Recovery Treatment Center to help addicted players recover. He has put John Lucas Fitness Systems into seven Houston hospitals to help drug-dependent young people and adults. And he has established the anti-drug group, STAND—"Students Taking Action, Not Drugs." Through STAND, groups of kids get together once a week. They don't talk about drug problems. They talk about "living" problems—things that have happened to them that make them feel worried, or ashamed, or jealous, or sad, or lonely. They talk about how to cope with feelings of anger and failure. They learn how to accept themselves for who they are. They learn how to be proud of themselves.

Athletes like Carl Eller, Spencer Haywood, Derek Sanderson, and John Lucas know that saying "No" to drugs isn't always easy. They know that kids will see other people taking drugs. They know that kids will read about famous athletes taking drugs. They know that kids may feel peer pressure to try drugs or be tempted to use drugs as an escape. And they know that saying "No" to drugs *today* may not stop a kid from trying drugs *tomorrow.*

"What makes drugs and alcohol so tough a problem," says John Lucas, "is that some people think a kid can say 'No' to drugs one time, and that it will last for life." But Lucas knows that the drug problem doesn't work that way:

> *"There are so many outside forces. It's kind of like getting your car washed once a week. One wash won't make your car clean forever. You have to say 'No' to drugs every day, every time a new problem comes up."*

Over and over, athletes say these things to young people. They try to help young people find *healthy* ways to solve the problems in sports. They try to help young people find *healthy* ways to solve the problems in life. And they have some very good advice:

- Believe in yourself, and take the time to be proud of who and what you are. Don't make sports—or any other interest—your whole life. Develop other interests, too.

- Work hard at being the best athlete and the best person you can be. But don't feel like a failure if you miss a free throw, fumble a ball, or strike out. Come back tomorrow and try again.

- When the game is over, go forward into the rest of your day, the rest of your life. Be a whole person. Talk to other people. You'll find out that they have problems that are similar to yours. Work together to find good answers.

- Find someone you can trust—a parent, a teacher, a doctor. Talk and listen.

- Take care of your body. If you're an athlete, work hard; but you don't need to over-train. Remember that your body is still growing. Eat well-balanced meals and get plenty of rest.

- Never try to solve problems by taking drugs. The problems don't go away for long. And drugs will just make all the other problems worse. Then drugs will become your worst problem of all.

If there is one best solution to the drug problem—in sports and out of sports—it lives within each athlete and each one of us. It lives within our feelings of pride and self-esteem—of "feeling good" about ourselves. It's acceptance of who we are and our willingness to accept the fact of losing—a contest, a game, a school election, a prize—without losing our sense of being winners as people.

"If you accept yourself the way you are," John Lucas says, "and then someone says, 'You need a drink to feel good,' you can say, 'Well, I feel good about myself already.'"

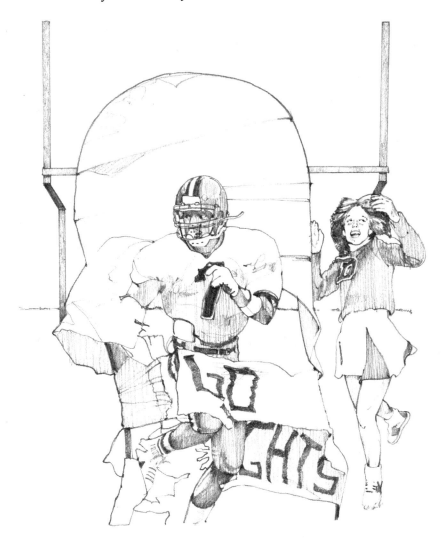

The solution also lives within our ability to make good decisions. Derek Sanderson says:

"You always have two choices—yes or no, right or wrong, good or evil. You make the decision. I'm not saying the world's going to be an easy place. You may have a tough go of it. But you go out and do the right thing. That will be the way to get pride. That will be the way to get peace of mind."

Taking drugs is a bad decision. Drugs are often taken as a solution to a problem that seems too big to solve any other way. But there *are* other ways. And the solution to the drug problem lies in finding ways to be and do your best—without drugs.

Each one of us can make the decision to work hard to find those ways.

Each one of us can make the decision to say "No" to drugs.

Glossary

addiction	the constant need or craving for a drug
alcohol	a depressant drug found in beer, wine, and liquor
amphetamine	one of several kinds of stimulant drugs
anabolic steroids	a group of synthetic male hormones sometimes used to enhance sports performance
beta-blocker	one kind of drug that helps control stress
cocaine	a stimulant drug made from the coca plant
crack	a form of cocaine made to be smoked
dependence	when a person needs drugs to avoid feeling sick
depressant	a drug that slows down the way the brain works
diuretic	a drug that flushes water out of the body
gateway drug	a drug that may lead to the use of other drugs
human growth hormone	a natural chemical that regulates body growth; sometimes used as a performance-enhancing drug
marijuana	a drug made from the cannabis, or hemp, plant
peer pressure	the feeling that you have to do something because other people are doing it
performance-enhancing drug	a drug used by an athlete to help improve sports performance
psychoactive drug	a drug that changes the way the brain works
roid rage	violent behavior caused by anabolic steroids
stimulant	a drug that speeds up the way the brain works
testosterone	the body's natural male hormone
tolerance	when the body and brain need more and more of a drug to get the same effects
withdrawal	the sick feeling addicts get when they stop taking the drugs they are dependent on

Index